Prepping and Survival Guide

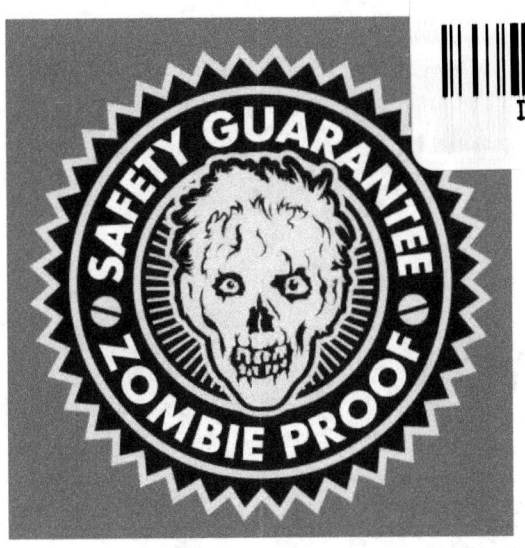

Are You Prepared for the

Zombie Apocalypse?

Prepping and Survival Series

Mendon Cottage Books

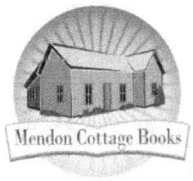

JD-Biz Publishing

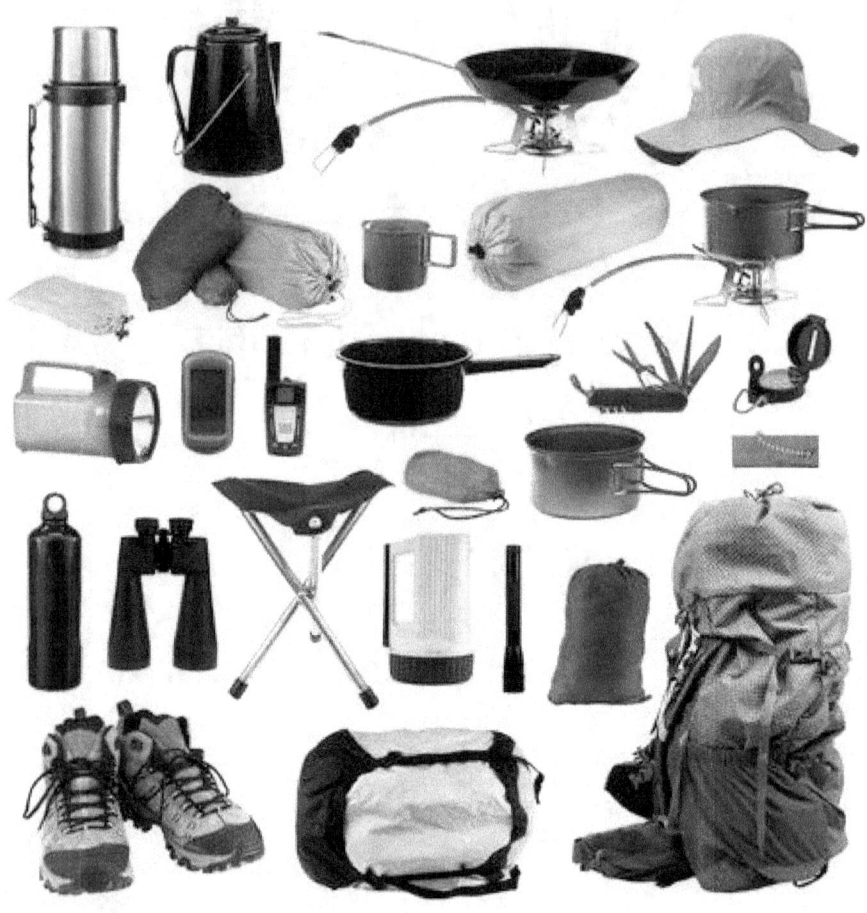

Table of Contents

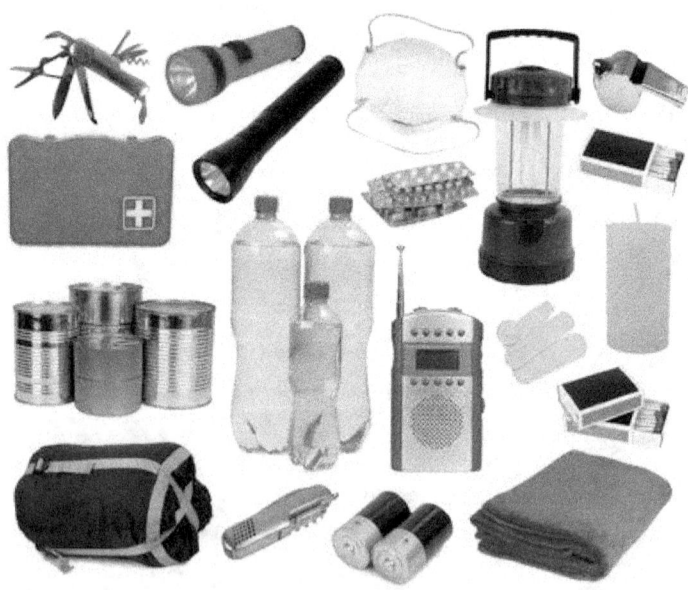

Introduction:

Not so long ago people considered prepping for unexpected events and catastrophes as behavior characterized as paranoid, over cautious and in some situations even mentally unstable. However, knowledge and awareness has advanced people's thinking over time about being proactive towards emergencies and disasters. Today there are special courses and training programs that teach the general public how to be prepared for any disaster or unforeseen events.

Ranging from hurricanes, floods, earthquakes, forest fires to bomb explosions, getting lost in the wilderness, economic crisis, accidents and medical emergencies all types of disasters need a management plan. Such a plan cannot only reduce the impact of the respective disaster but at times can even prevent it from happening. It also gives the victims a stronger sense of confidence and patience.

Surviving difficult circumstances is a natural human instinct and with the increase in awareness and knowledge, this instinct is also getting stronger. Over the years, the survival and endurance qualities have not only increased but in some scenarios, they have also changed altogether. With more advancement in technology, people have become very dependent on the utility elements of society like electricity, water supplies, heating and cooling systems and other forms of machinery. Day to day life is more and more dependent on daily appliances like blenders, vacuum cleaners, mobile phones, computers, electric blankets, torches, battery operated equipment and the list goes on. Survival without these in normal circumstances can become cumbersome and difficult. They have become necessities of life.

So it is of utmost importance that we be knowledgeable of the basic survival techniques and skills and minimize the impact of unforeseen or disastrous events by being prepped for the worst. If these things are deeply embedded in our minds and our lifestyles, it will automatically make this world a safer place to live in.

The key factors that affect human behaviors in this context are the various circumstances that they face. All events and disasters vary from situational factors. Analyzing the risk of a situation and then dealing with it in a systematic way is the right path to follow. The main thing to do here is to self-assess before preparing for the outside. What will be your reactions and actions in such situations? How will your body behave? Assess your capabilities and skills before actually chalking out a plan for prepping and survival. Where do you need training? What are your strengths and weaknesses? Survival is the application of some basic techniques and principles and their adaptation to the various situations.

The three basic factors that trigger the instinct for survival and prepping in humans are:

The fear of losing your life and loved ones

The knowledge of what is needed to survive

The possession of equipment needed to fight a disaster

Hence, the quest for knowledge and the effort to survive anywhere in the world will never end at any given point. This guidebook helps identify some key prepping and survival principles and strategies.

What to Prep For:

The first question that you must ask before you start prepping and survival planning is what disasters or events could happen to endanger your safety and survival. The reality is that it is not possible to prepare for everything. Experts suggest that one should prepare for potential disasters or events that might occur in the next 4-5 years. This does not mean that you undermine the preparedness phenomenon; it is only a way to make it a little more convenient and humane.

So how to plan?

Take some time out and sit and think.

Do some brainstorming.

Predict what might happen in the next five years around you.

Research newspapers, articles and the internet

Talk with people.

Have a look around your house. See what the potential threat sources are within a five- mile radius. Is there any danger of flooding or drought? Is there a nuclear plant or dam in the vicinity?

Evaluate weather conditions and trends like hurricanes, tsunami, earthquakes, storms, tornadoes, etc.

Are there any warning systems?

Be pessimistic and analyze the situation.

After you have penned down these answers, you need to create a chart about the potential hazards or disasters and the adverse effects they might have on you and your family. The following is a sample chart of the same sort with some examples for illustrations:

Potential Disaster or Expected Event	Adverse Outcomes
For Example: *Storms with heavy rains and power outage*	Food will be Spoiled No heating or cooling systems Blockage of roads and streets due to falling trees and poles Mild flooding danger

	Breakdown of communication lines and transportation facilities Lightening striking trees can cause fire
Snow storms and blizzards	Power outage Heating impairment Frozen pipes and water shortage Blocked communication Food shortage and unavailability of supplies
Civil disorders or riots in city	• Blockage of roads and links • Stranded without food and water • Inability to reach family and home • Potential theft or looting threats • Fire and shoot out
Vehicle breakdown on a wilderness expedition	• Stranded without communication • Shortage of food and supplies • Danger from wild life

	• Adverse weather conditions
	• Unavailability of shelter and protection

Once you have outlined your potential risks and hazards you will be in a better situation to decide about your future modus operandi.

Important Decision for Survival:

The basic decision that one must make in all scenarios is to fight the circumstances, remain safe and wait for rescue. There are pros and cons of both. After weighing the advantages and disadvantages, one must decide whether or not to execute the evacuation plan of the disaster. Once you have decided to execute, there will be no turning. The evacuation plan should answer the following questions:

Where to Go?

Decide on a location for evacuation. It is important to list down some options that are most viable and easy to approach. The location should be such that the effects of the disaster should not harshly hit you there. The best way is to coordinate in advance with friends or relatives living in a safer place. This safe location can be in the near vicinity or 100 to 200 miles away depending on the magnitude of the disaster. Some important guidelines in this regard are as follows:

> The disaster or adverse conditions that you are facing should not be prevalent at that place or vice versa. This way your location can be a safe house for someone else when they need it for evacuation.

> Must chalk out the routes and alternatives

> Decide the evacuation mode i.e. by foot, car or public transport.

Ensure maintenance of the evacuation vehicle, arrange for spare tires, and reserve fuel.

Keeping into consideration hotels and guesthouses is a good choice. Seek prior information about their boarding and lodging charges and terms and conditions.

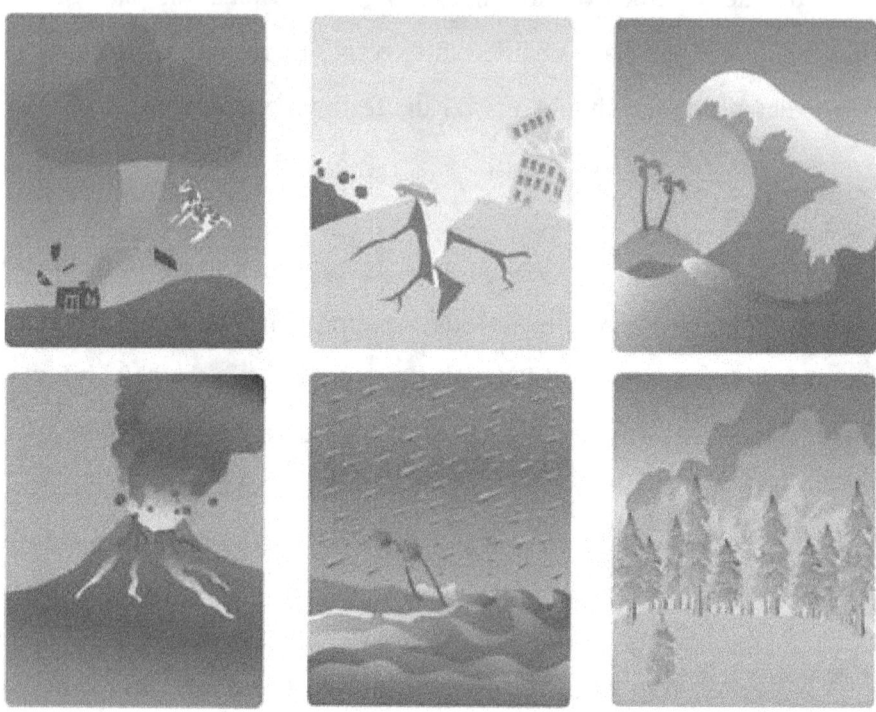

How to Get There and What to Carry?

This section covers the ultimate survival and prepping basics, which might be needed, while travelling on a journey or towards a safer place.

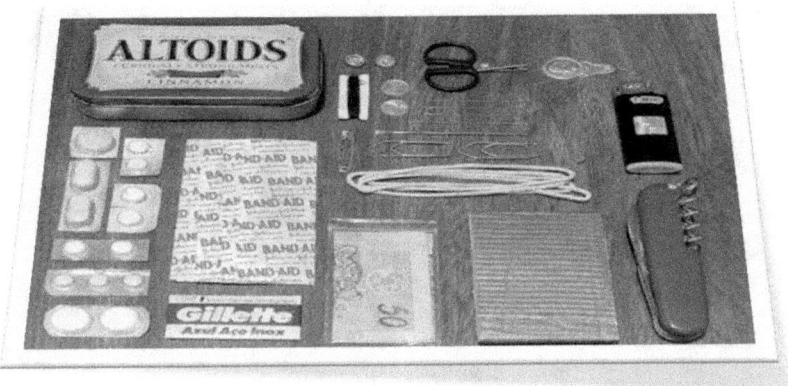

Basics for Prepping and Survival:

The first and the foremost attention should be given to the preparation phase of the process. This means that you should assess the current situation and identify the need for the right apparatus and survival equipment. Not only should one focus on the physical equipment but also preparing the human aspects of psychology, emotions and personal health is of vital importance. Being prepared to cope with different levels of stress and anxiety and dealing with adverse conditions has to be top most priority of a survivor.

Prepping:

The principle to keep in mind before starting a journey or a plan for survival is to undergo the following phases:

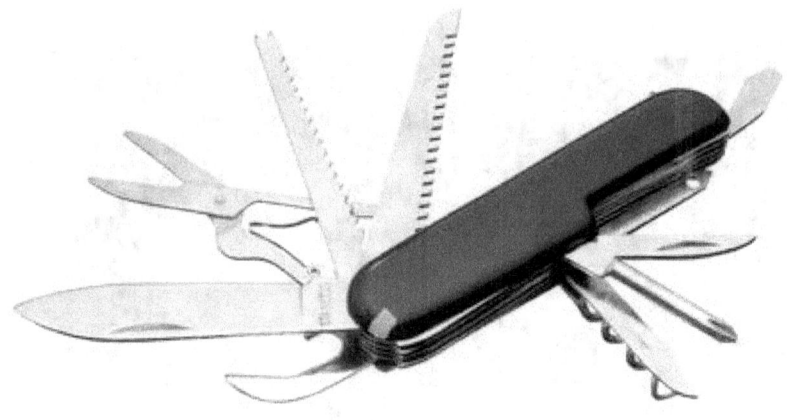

Being Prepared for Different Situations:

The motto of the Boy Scouts, "Be Prepared", is the essence of resisting and fighting any disaster or mishap.

Analyze the Conditions and Gather Information:

If someone is planning to go on a journey or starting some sort of survival planning, the first step is to gain as much information about the place and situation as possible. The larger quantity of information will help assess the conditions of the place and identify the likely problems that one might face while going through this process.

Need Assessment:

The next process is to identify what survival equipment and gadgets are in hand, and what additional help or equipment might be needed in such a situation. Some of the important questions that one can consider before analyzing may include:

What will be the duration of the trip or situation?

How much edibles and food items will be consumed during that period?

How much water will be required during that period?

What will be the weather conditions and what kinds of clothes will be essential?

What kind of shoes might be required and what kind of terrain will be present?

Any special equipment or machinery that might be required for that terrain

What medical problems can occur during that journey or trip?

Survival Kit Development:

Development of a good survival kit is essential for success. Some important considerations before assembling the kit:

List down what is needed and what is not.

Make a checklist to avoid mistakes.

Don't make the kit to heavy or large.

Make sure all equipment being carried is in running condition and not out dated or expired.

Must be easy to carry with handles or straps

Must have a first aid box

Medical Checks:

Before you start any journey, you must have a medical check up to assess your health conditions and fitness levels. Even if there is no journey planned, regular medical checkups enable a person to timely detect any malfunctions of organs or prevent other alarming medical conditions. It is also important to keep some common over the counter medicines and first aid supplies on hand to cope with any small emergencies.

It is also important to follow a proper vaccination plan to overcome the threats and risks of catching any viral or bacterial diseases like yellow fever, cholera, tetanus, meningitis, diphtheria and typhoid fever. If suffering from any kind of medical problem, the medicines pertaining to that disease must in hand to maintain health.

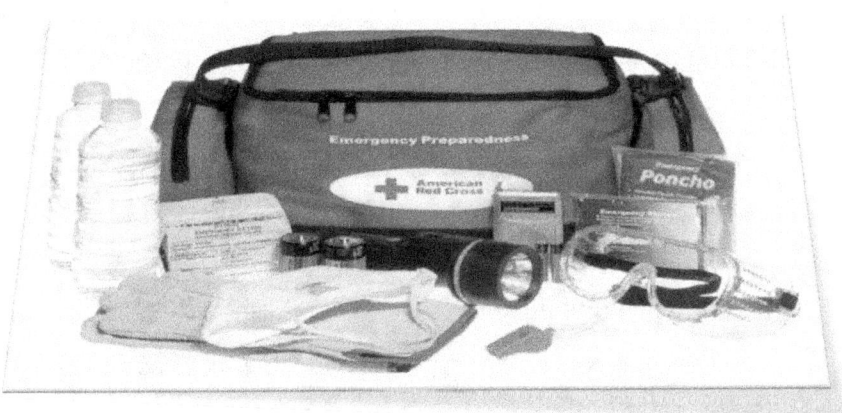

Carryout Effective Research:

Gathering information about natural disasters or any journey or place that you are planning to visit is an essential part of the prepping process. The more information you have the better you are able to understand the conditions and scenarios of the situation. Effective methods of carrying out the research involve the following:

Contacting people who have already gone through such circumstances or living in those places. They are best source of information because they have themselves encountered and faced such problems and scenarios.

Reading books written about the respective place or terrain is an important research method. A great number of books are available in the market not only about specific disasters, events or places but also about general prepping tips and techniques.

Online research is the latest methodology for prepping. There are dedicated websites, blogs and magazines available that can guide you about various situations and latest equipment that may act very helpful.

For better prepping for survival one should take up survival trainings and courses that provide valuable information about:

- how to build shelters and makeshift arrangements for living in different situations

- how to find water and store it

- methods of finding food sources and types of wild foods

- fire building techniques and tips

- knowledge about herbal healthcare treatment and first aid

Map reading and acquiring the related maps is important if going out on a journey or trip. Maps may also be important in general if in a disaster you want to locate emergency services of police, rescue, hospital or any other important building. It can also indicate alternative routes and roads.

Carryout Effective Planning before Actual Execution:

Planning is an organized method of preparing for an event in a systemic way. It requires careful analysis of the needs, requirements and expected conditions of the event. Plans may vary according to the circumstances of different situations. Following are some guidelines that should be followed to create a good plan:

Create a logical sequence of events. A flow chart in this regard is quite effective.

Divide the journey or event into project phases like entry, goals and objectives, potential risks, stimuli, execution and rescue and recovery.

Chalk out a survival plan.

Identify various small tasks to complete various phases.

Ensure that roles and responsibilities are delegated according various tasks that need to be accomplished food collector, driver, medical advisor, navigator, cook, mechanic, equipment supplier, etc.

Device charts to monitor progress on various steps according to time and supplies.

Keep room for natural calamities and unforeseen mishaps like breakdowns, medical problems, breakage, etc.

Chalk out alternative routes.

Make sure that all participants are involved. Everyone in the prepping and planning process should be aware of the plan and always leave contact information at the rear base camp.

There should always be a contingency plan with everyone.

Before starting any expedition or journey, tell people where you are going and how long you will take to get back. Therefore, in case of foul play, someone might get worried and initiate a search and rescue operation.

Supplies and Equipment for Survival:

Prepping the equipment and supplies is an important part of the process. As already established in the initial phases, what will be the needs of the event, here a detailed look into the equipment requirement is carried out. Depending upon whether you are on foot or travelling by vehicle, list down the most reliable, easy to carry equipment that will meet the required needs with efficiency and effectiveness.

Keeping into view the research done in early phases and the information and data collected, the following aspects of survival equipment should be considered in general:

Cash or Checks:

Before leaving your house, make sure you have at least $1000 more or less depending on the distance you are planning on travelling. Keeping smaller bills can be convenient at various locations. Travelers' checks can also be a good option for long journeys.

Duplicate Documents:

Have a duplicate set of important documents always ready for your move. This may include ID, Social Security Card, bank documents or passport. You should also have a list of phone numbers and contacts for emergency situations.

Clothes Needed for Survival:

The right choice of clothing can save human beings from a lot of natural problems and illnesses. Depending upon the climate of the region, the time of event and the bodily properties of the individual, selection or clothes should be made with care. In colder climates, jackets and jerseys should be available and while in tropical regions, airy and cool clothes should be arranged. It should not be forgotten that a spare set of clothing is needed if some problem or mishap occurs.

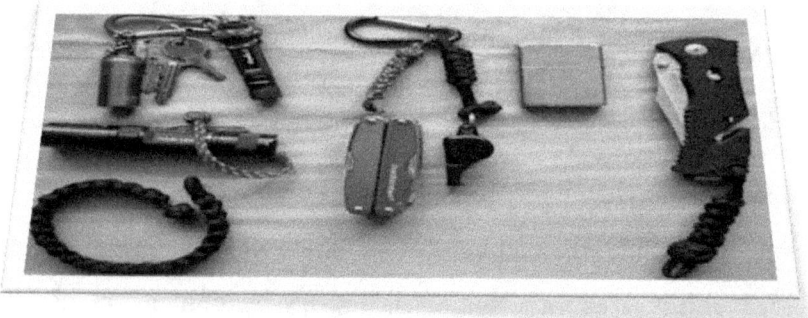

Another important aspect to consider is that clothes should be both comfortable and at the same time practical according to the needs of the event. One should avoid using heavy clothing when you have to walk or engage in some sort of physical activity. They should not be very flashy or conspicuous. The material should be easy to dry and if required, waterproof should be preferred. Whatever you select to wear should be well fitted and not loose or hanging. It should provide some level of protection from the adverse and harsh effects of climate like sunlight, wind, snow, rain or any other natural weather conditions. However, proper ventilation is a must to keep the body fresh and energetic. Breathable materials like Gore-Tex are a very good option for tropical climates. The color of the clothes is also an important consideration.

Wearing the appropriate shoes suitable for the respective activity or terrain is very important. If you have to walk, climb, or have a foot intensive activity that needs to be carried out, you must select shoes according to the requirement. Comfort, ease of wearing, reliability and durability are the key aspects that need to be kept in mind. Make sure that shoes have already been worn beforehand so that if there is a problem with the fit, you might fix it before the event. However, don't over emphasize this as clothes are only clothes. There are worse things that can happen.

Sleeping Mats and Bags:

Taking adequate and comfortable rest while in harsh situations or during a journey is very critical for survival. Therefore carrying a sleeping bag or mat to rest on is very important. Generally, there are two varieties of bags available in the market. One is hollow filled with synthetic fibers while the second style is filled with down. Down is a very effective filling material that keeps the bag light and strengthens its insulation properties. Keeping these bags away from water is of utmost importance for them to remain effective.

Back Packs and Bags:

Depending upon the conditions and activities involved in the survival situation, it is important to assess the need for luggage. How will items be carried from one place to another? What should be the size and weight to carried easily? Keeping these considerations in mind, one must select a strong, reliable backpack that is comfortable and not burdensome. It should accommodate all your survival gear and at the same time keep it safe and protected. There is no point of carrying damaged equipment. The material of the backpack and its structure can make all the difference. In addition, your way of carrying it and lifting it is also very critical for long journeys on foot. It should have many pockets to segment things according to needs.

Packing or Stowing:

To avoid materials and supplies from getting wet one can use a polyethene cover or packing. The supplies should be packed in the backpack in such an organized way that searching for any equipment does not affect or obstruct the actions. Some important guidelines in this regard are as follows:

Keep the tent at the very top so that the first step of tent erection can be done before any other action.

Sleeping bags can be at the extreme bottom.

Heavy equipment and luggage should be placed at the bottom as well.

Cooking utensils should be aligned at the sides so that during short breaks these can be used without unpacking other things.

Food items should be carefully placed according to needs and their perish ability. They should be placed in proper hard airtight containers that are not prone to leakage during the travel.

Ration the supplies according the needs of the traveler.

Global Positioning System:

Benefiting from the most advanced form of technology in the prepping and survival field is use of GPS or global positioning system. This is a technical gadget, which helps identify your position anywhere in the world by sending and receiving satellite signals. The device has reduced the need for a navigator or locator in a survival journey. It is very user friendly and is up to 95% accurate in its results. However, like all technology gadgets it also has a limited life and serviceability. So use of maps should not be eliminated.

Radios and Cell Phones:

For a very long time, radio has been a basic survival and communication tool for remote areas and expeditions. However just having the radio is not enough; the ability to use it effectively is also a key consideration. Before going on a journey or to the wilderness one must learn its channeling, tuning and transmission functions. To be more prepared, there should be prearrangement about regular transmissions and a set schedule.

Another similar invention is the use of mobile phones. Where radio is difficult to use, heavy mobile phones are better options for smaller journeys. However, here the limitation of charging and restricted battery life and serviceability is unavoidable.

Altimeters and Compasses:

These navigational tools are very useful when going to mountainous areas and hill stations.

Survival Kit:

Having appropriate survival goods on hand is important to the success of the evacuation process. Whether you are out to find your safe house or on a planned journey into the wilderness, the survival kit is a must for all. Make a list of all the things that might be required along the way and keep them in a small tight box for safety. Some important components of a survival kit may include the following:

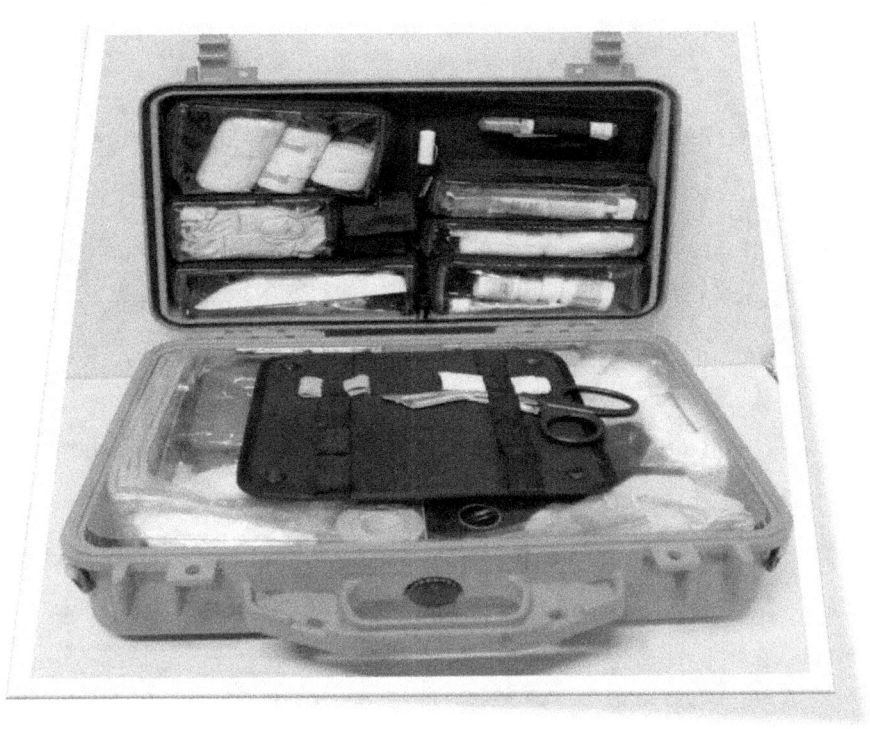

Matches or Lighters are a must for all survival kits. As already explained, there are five basic components of survival and fire is one of them. This fire can be created easily if you have a matchbox or lighter available. Preventing matches from getting wet is very important. Also, use them wisely and don't waste them. Keeping a flint in reserve is also a good option. They even work in wet conditions thus increasing effectiveness.

Candles and Torches are essential elements if travelling at night. Even if not during a disaster, anything can happen and you may have to take darker pathways. For such purposes you must have a candle and good quality flash lights.

Needle and Thread is very useful for unforeseen tears and breakages. Having different sized needles is a wiser option ranging from very large to small. They can not only be useful in sewing clothes but also tents, sleeping bags, shoes and any other element needing repairs. The threads should also be strong and durable.

Fishing Hooks and Lines are needed for food emergencies. When you have a food shortage and a fish source is available, use of fishhook and line to catch some prey can save lives. These can also be used for making traps for other smaller animals like squirrels or birds.

Magnifying Glass can be used for both starting a fire and observing minute objects.

Snare Wire is a multi-purpose material that can be used in several ways. Depending on the situation, its utility can be a great advantage to human beings.

Beta Lights are coin sized illuminated objects that can stay functional for more than a decade. They are non-battery operated and can very useful in emergencies and dark situations.

Signal Flares are a basic survival kit component. While travelling for long distances and in the wilderness, these can exponentially aid search and rescue operations. However, you must learn how to operate one of these prior to the disaster. In addition, they should be stored carefully because they are explosive materials and can cause significant harm if misused.

Markers are good for labeling things and using arrows or other signals to point out your location or path.

Brewing Components like milk powder sachets, tea bags and instant coffee, sugar and sweeteners. These are a good morale booster and help one remain fresh and active. Every now and then, a small tea break can help revive energies and efforts.

Survival Food Items are a must to keep on living. You might not necessarily be looking to get fat but keeping up the calorie count is what is important. You can stock your survival kit with the essentials like butter tubes, ghee, dehydrated meat, chocolates, salt and pepper and other forms of canned or survival foods available in packs in the markets.

Knives and Blades are vital for any trip whether planned or unplanned. Carry a small sized multi-purpose knife or a Swiss knife with folding capabilities. Surgical blades can also be useful in many circumstances. Make sure both are very sharp. If they need sharpening you should know the right methods to accomplish this beforehand.

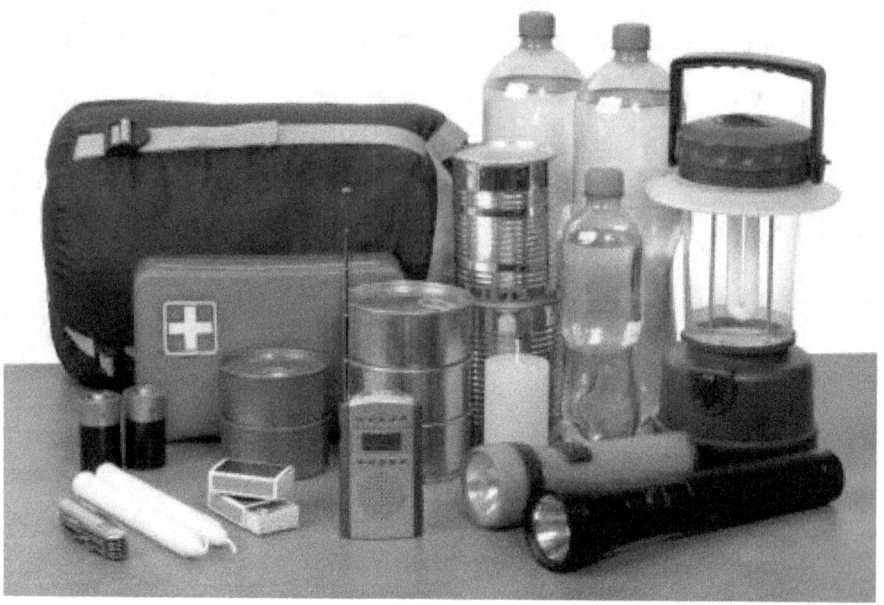

Five Essential Survival Skills:

Survival skills may involve a cumulative knowledge and learning capabilities of various methodologies and strategies, and techniques that may be required in adverse circumstances. They are mostly needed when modern day luxuries and facilities are not available or have been broken down. In general, survival skills are mostly considered in context of being in the wild outside but in reality may be effective in all kinds of survival endeavors. It may range from a wide variety of options and choices but the five basic and most essential skills for survival are:

Shelter and Protection:

Whether you are in the middle of any disaster or unplanned event, protecting yourself from the adversities of the surrounding and environment is a must for survival. Direct exposures to harsh conditions can have serious outcomes. Therefore, if you are in a survival situation, building and finding an appropriate shelter is an essential skill that is needed. Important guidelines in this regard are:

Proactively learn how to build different kinds of shelters from limited resources and materials.

Select shelter based on weather conditions, location, safety levels, light sources, etc.

The size of the shelter should be in accordance with the number of participants.

There are many types of shelters to choose from. There can be naturally formed shelters like caves, large hollow trees and logs or they can be made according to needs like mud huts, tents, snow shelters, and shrub or tree huts.

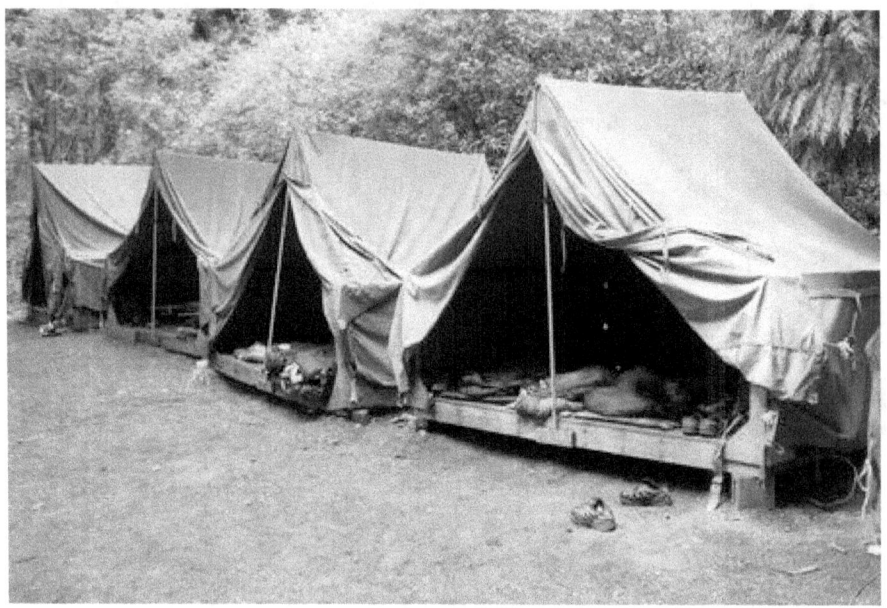

Water:

Water is an essential component of the human body. It may not only be required for drinking but for carrying out various everyday chores as well. From washing to cooking, water is needed in most activities and is a must for survival. Meeting the water needs of human being is very important. Depending on weather conditions, the requirement of water may be more or less but it will never end.

Anyone preparing for survival training should learn how to find water sources and how to store and use water accordingly. Clean water for drinking purposes can be obtained from springs, morning dew, rain or rivers and streams. In a survival situation, you may also need to purify or clean the water yourself. So be prepared. Use effective and efficient methods including the addition of chemicals like iodine, filtration process, or boiling. You must also be aware of herbal treatments for water purification. In certain circumstances, you must also learn how to store water.

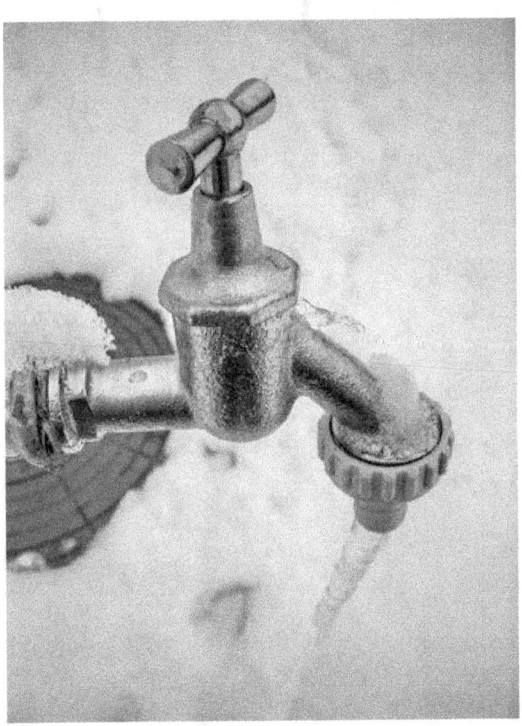

Fire:

If you have a survival kit with a matchbox or lighter, it's a survival blessing, but if not then you must be prepared for the worst. Just like water is an essential for survival so is fire. Building a fire can be difficult if you don't know how. Go for proactive training about learning how to start fires from limited resources. Learn about basic combustion materials and their utility. It is not only important for cooking or keeping warm but also for creating a protective perimeter against many dangers.

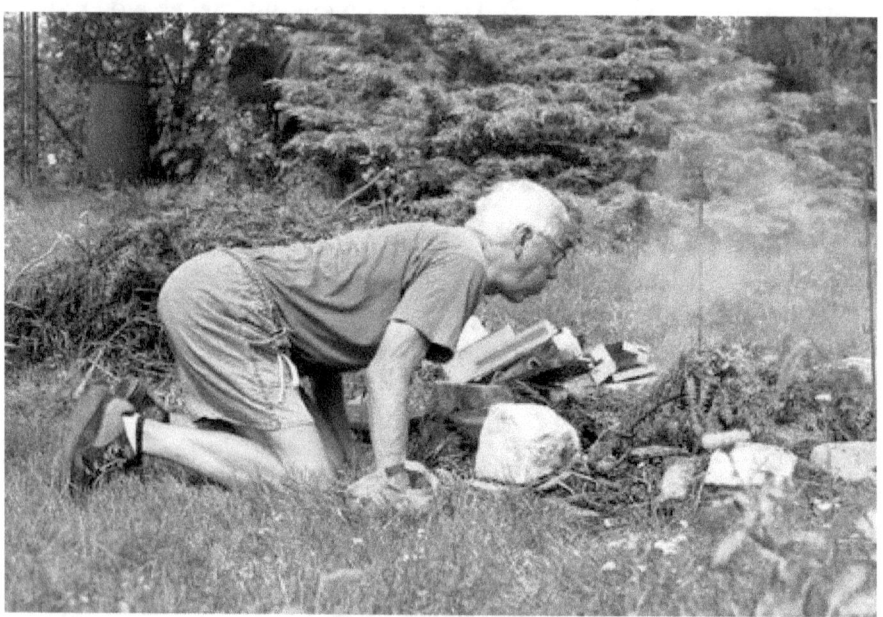

Food:

No living being can survive without food. Update your knowledge about food requirements and nutritional properties of things. Learn how to make the maximum out of the minimum. Find natural sources of food. Learn basic hunting and preying tactics and skills.

Attitude:

Last but not the least one must keep up a positive attitude with the will to survive and continue living. You should have the motivation, determination and strong willpower. Losing hope can weaken your strengths. So keep your morale up and strong.

These five skills can definitely play a critical role in the survival of a disaster victim.

Conclusion:

After a detailed analysis of the prepping and survival basics, it must be quite clear that prepping for unforeseen calamities and events is the right option if you want to reduce the adversities. The essence of the process is to be prepared for the worst. You cannot be enough overcautious and alert. Just like the motto of boy scouts "BE PREPARED". This should be the motto of every intelligent survivor. The effectiveness to success is to follow an organized and pre-decided approach with formal training in areas, which are weak. You should know your survival basics as anyone can undergo a disaster.

Author bio

Books are a great medium of sharing one's own experiences with the outer world, and enhancing the knowledge of the readers. With this same purpose, I, Sneha Agrawal share this write-up with my readers.

I am an MBA graduate from a top notch Business School of India, and have done specialization in marketing and finance stream. I also hold some work experience as a team leader, for one of the known Indian IT companies.

To live a successful life, one should always have the answers of a few questions, at any point in time and they are what, how and when; and I live my life in search of these answers.

Our books are available at

1. Amazon.com
2. Barnes and Noble
3. Itunes
4. Kobo
5. Smashwords
6. Google Play Books

Check out some of the other JD-Biz Publishing books

Gardening Series on Amazon

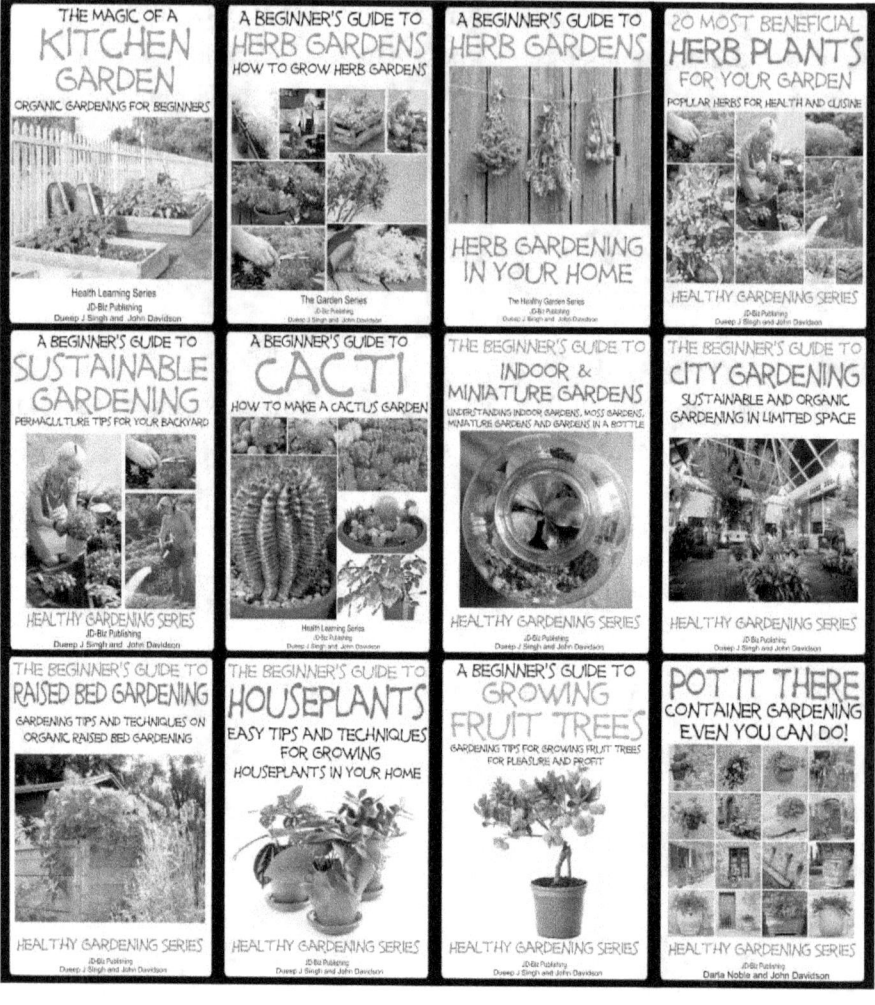

Health Learning Series

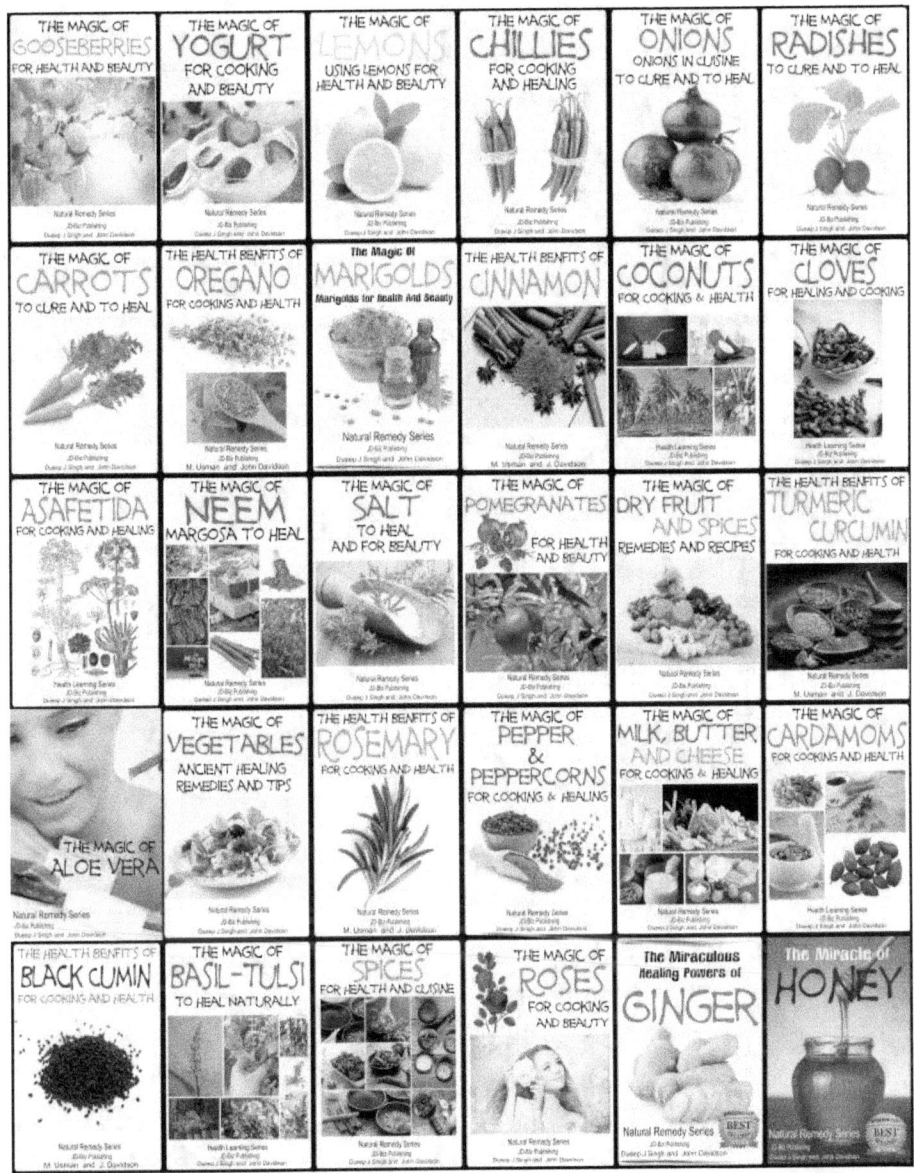

Country Life Books

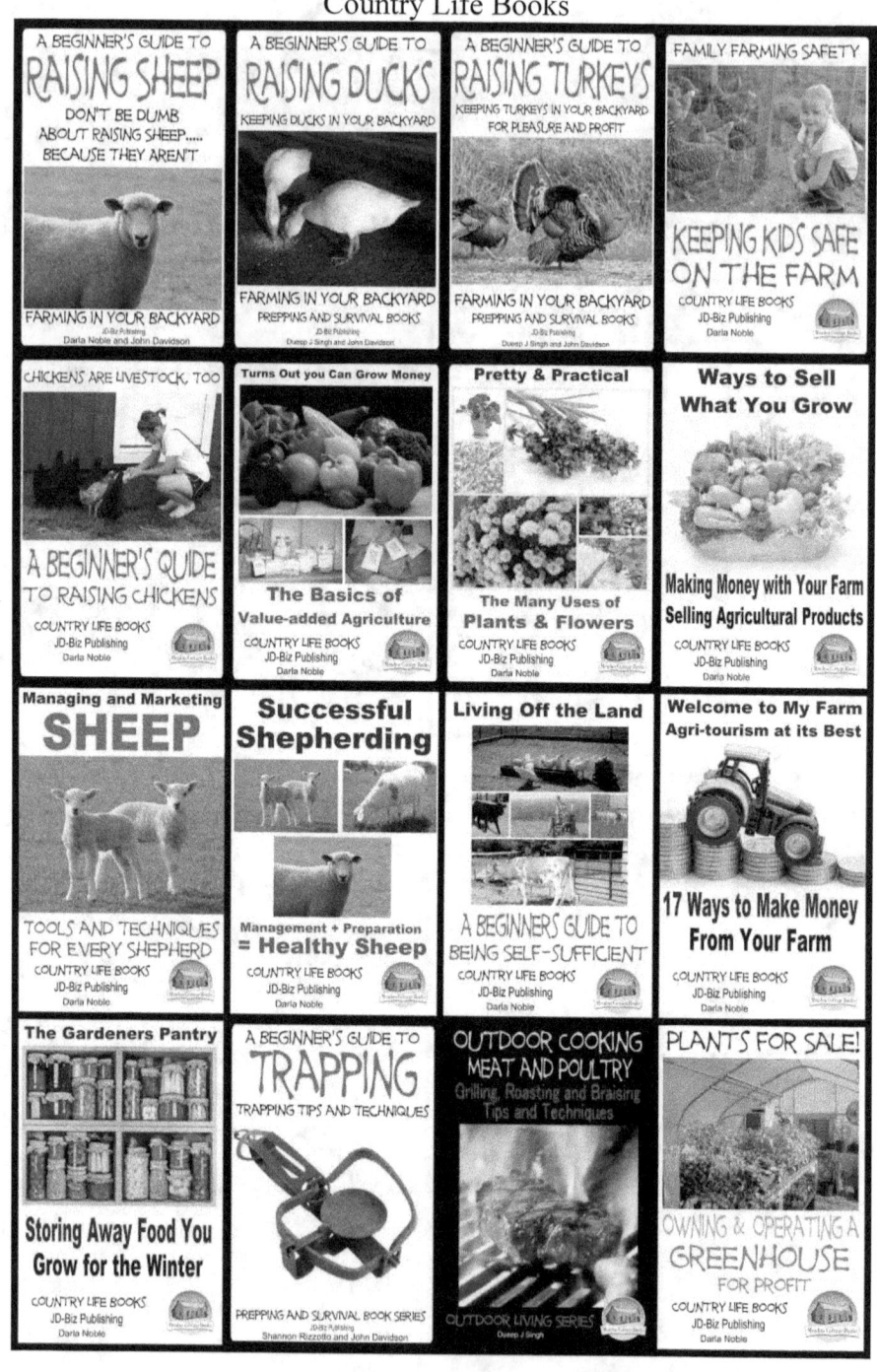

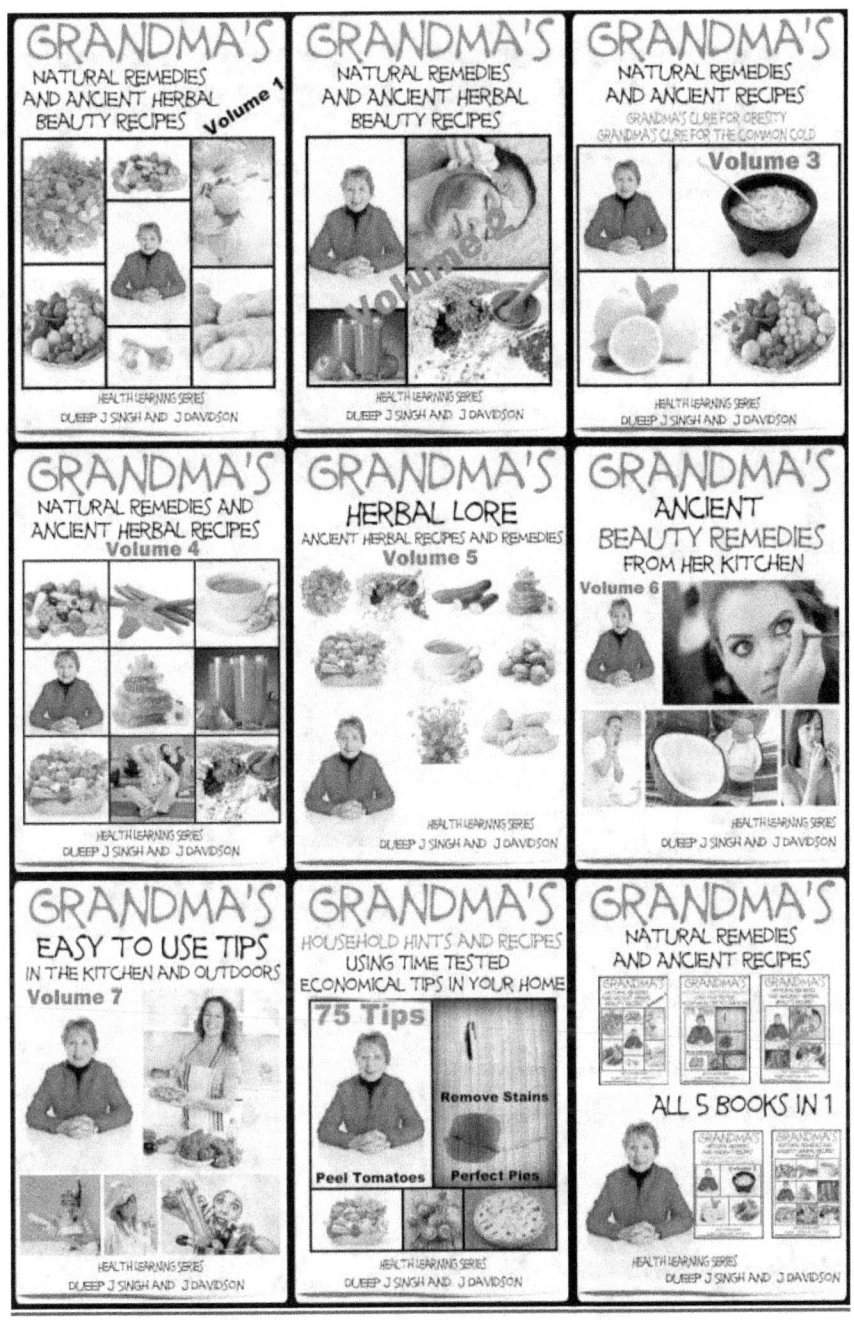

Health Learning Series

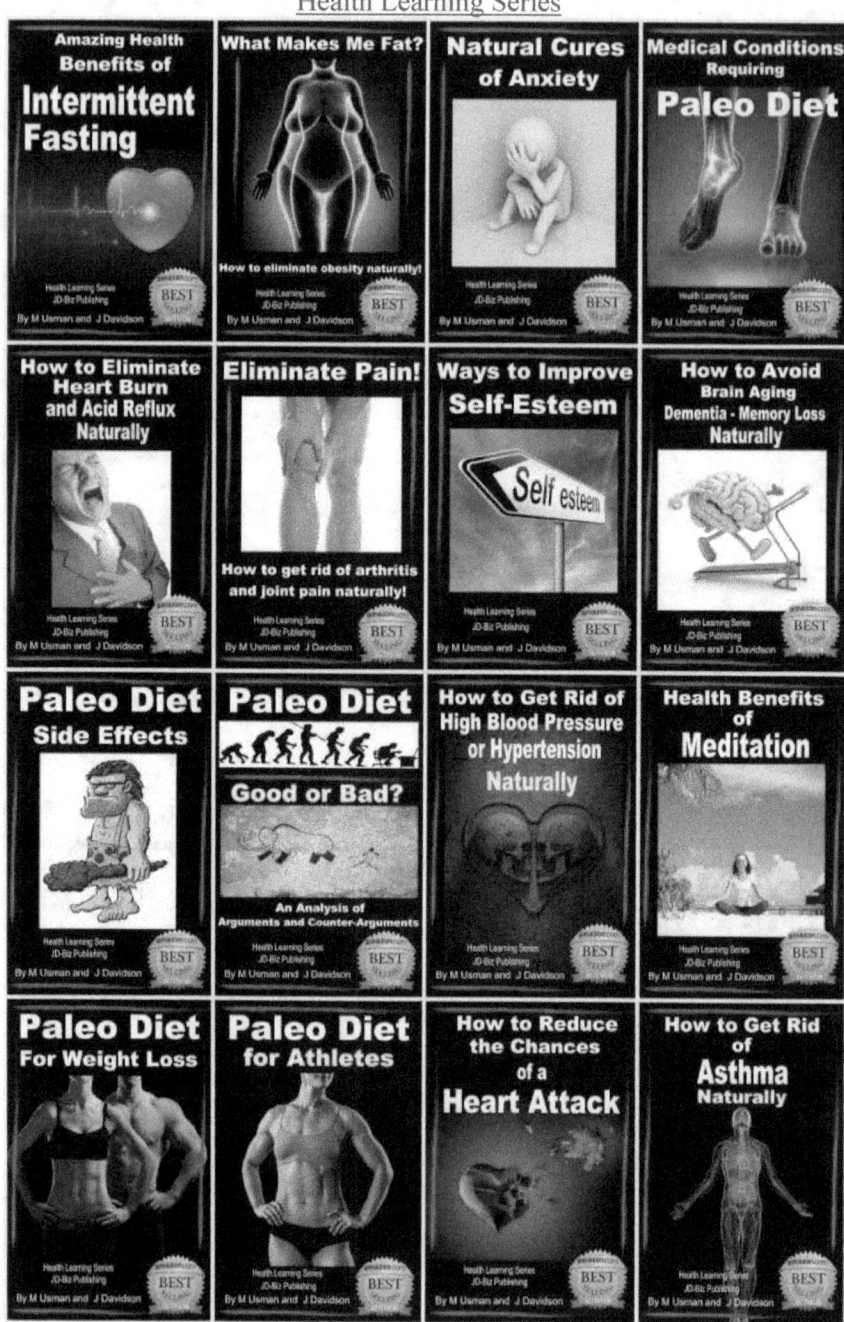

Amazing Animal Book Series

Learn To Draw Series

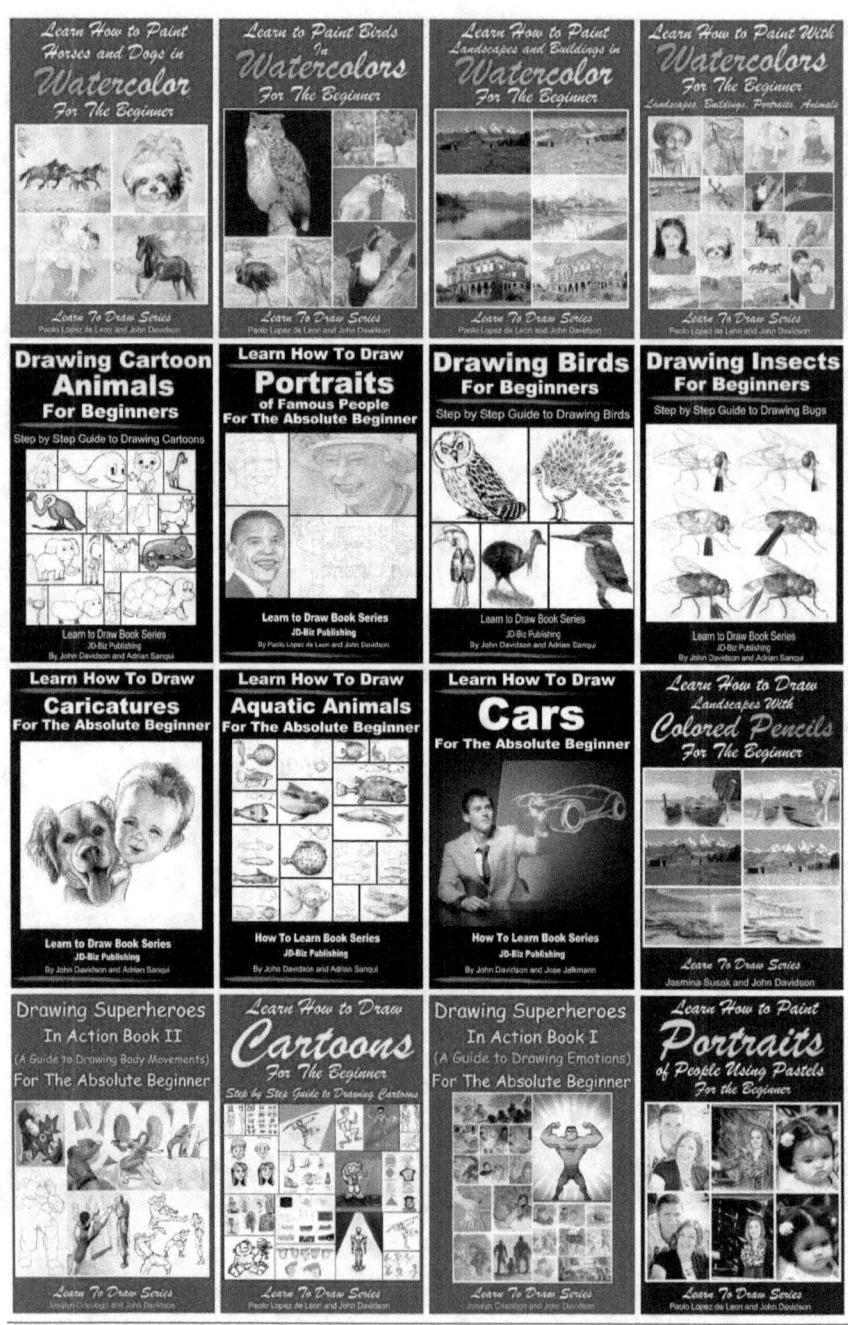

How to Build and Plan Books

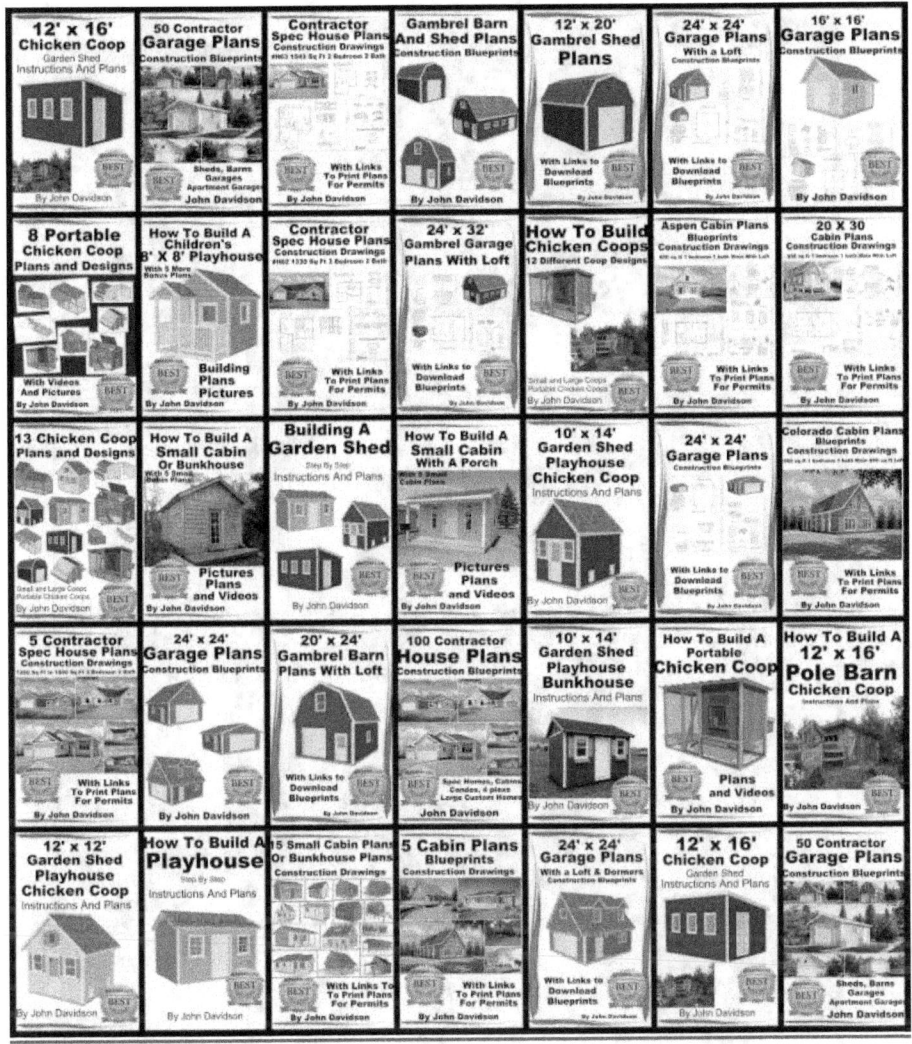

Entrepreneur Book Series

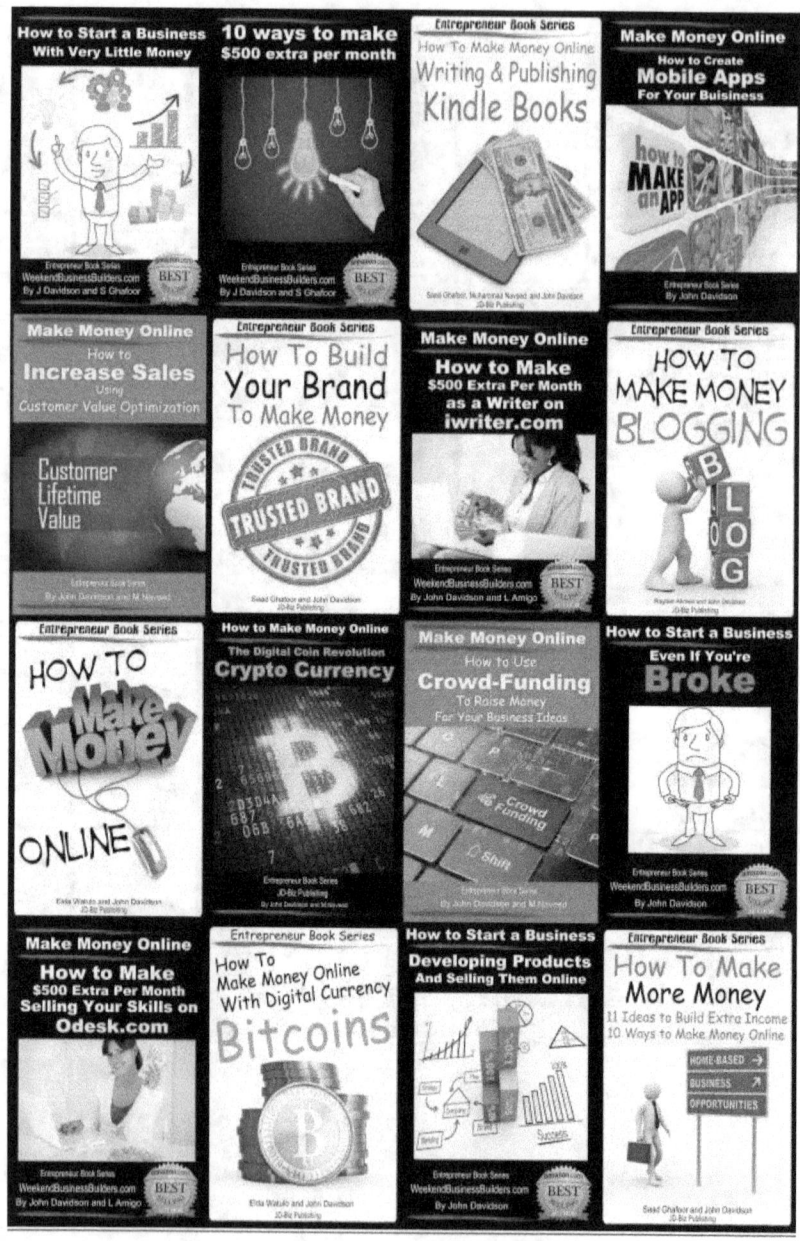

Publisher

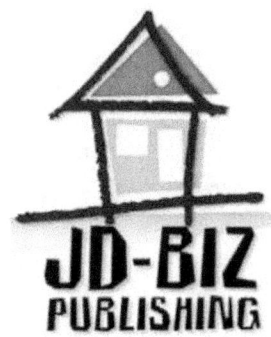

JD-Biz Corp

P O Box 374

Mendon, Utah 84325

http://www.jd-biz.com/

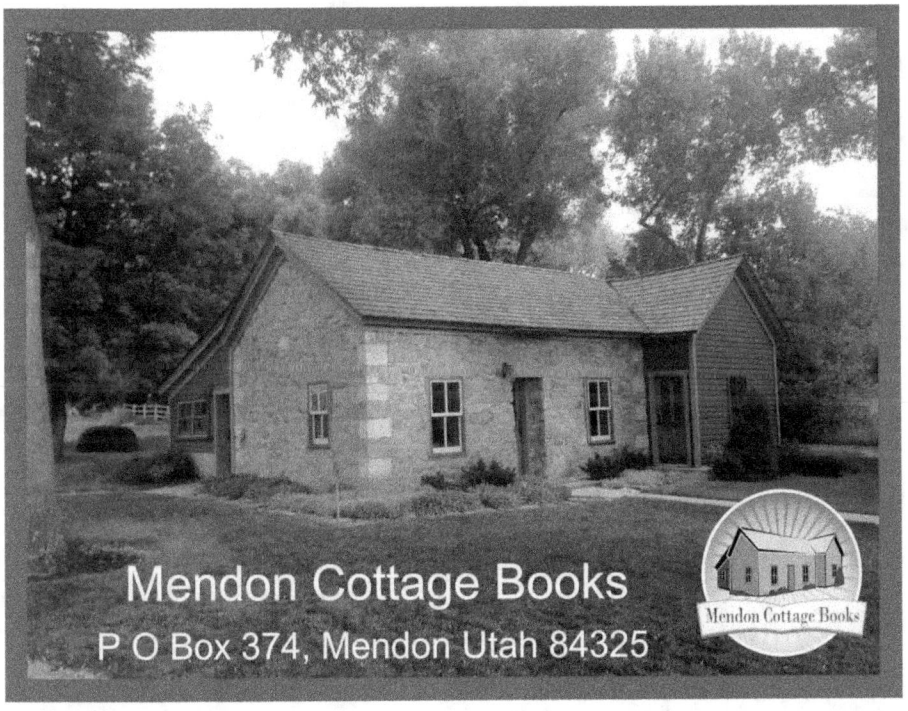